SAF
Essex*Works*.
For a better quality of life

D0513214

Angel's Quill Productions

30130 163392128

First Edition
© 2004 Mark Elliott Miller, MPH

Angel's Quill Productions
835 East Lamar Blvd., #357, Arlington, TX 76011
214-797-3197

Printed by
BooksJustBooks.com
51 East 42nd Street, Suite 1202, New York, NY 10017

Design and layout
Budget Book Design
9 Washington Avenue, Pleasantville, NY 10570

Library of Congress Catalog Number pending

ISBN: 0-9759516-0-2

Printed in the United States of America

CONTENTS

Other Titles By Mark Elliott Miller:

Extraordinary Encounters In An Ordinary Life
and
Advice For Life From The Mouths Of Elders,
One Hundred Ways To Grow Old Gracefully.
Available through all major bookstores and on-line at
www.iUniverse.com.

To my mother and father,
Louise and Hugh Miller,
for teaching me the true meaning of love.

FOREWORD

⁓

When my 47-year-old wife, Robyn, was diagnosed in May 2003 with multiple myeloma, a rare form of cancer of the bone marrow, our 10-year marriage changed forever. As a loving husband, there was never a question that I would do whatever was necessary to save my beloved wife's life. While I have worked in the health care industry since 1983 as a marketer and administrator, and I earned a Master of Public Health degree in 2000, no work experiences or education had prepared me for my soul mate's cancer.

By writing about my family's experiences with cancer, I found an effective way to get my feelings of fear and despair out in the open where they could be effectively managed. During my wife's battle with cancer, our family, friends, and coworkers were a great support emotionally and financially. Since we moved away from our Houston, Texas home to Arlington, Texas for Robyn to receive aggressive cancer care by Dr. Karel Dicke at the Arlington Cancer Center and Arlington Memorial Hospital, I sought a support group for husbands of women with cancer and found none. I wrote this book to provide assistance to other husbands of cancer patients. It is based on my career experiences and from observations made during my wife's treatments.

Ironically, as I wrote these words, I was figuratively walking in the well-worn shoes of my father, Hugh, on this journey. Fifteen years ago, his wife of 37-years and my mother, Louise, died in a Houston, Texas hospital after a long struggle with breast cancer that metastasized throughout her body. On February 28, 2004, one week after my father talked openly with me about finding the inner strength necessary to live through cancer, he died in a Houston nursing home. This book is dedicated to my parents. They embodied true love in good times and bad.

My mother's final words to my siblings and me were written on pages of a yellow legal pad while she lay in her hospital bed. She wrote of her pride in her children and shared her love one last time. As my mother gave comfort to her grieving five children, I hope this book will support husbands of cancer patients who have love in their hearts but are uncertain how to live with this dreaded disease in their families. A portion of profits from this book will be donated to cancer charities funding research. Research offers hope that our sons will have many healthy years to spend with their wives.

CHAPTER ONE

MAN VS. CANCER

❦

Your wife has cancer—undoubtedly the one illness that instills fear in the hearts of even the bravest men. From the moment you received the news, through the months or years of surgeries, chemotherapy and radiation therapy that follow, one phrase from your wedding vows will likely reverberate through your mind: "...in sickness and in health, 'til death do you part."

The fear of your wife's illness and her possible death—and your inability to control the situation—is overwhelming. As men, especially those of us raised in the Baby Boom generation, we were taught many clichés to handle any fastballs thrown across our plate.

"Be a man!"

"Do what you have to do!"

"Be strong for the family!"

"Keep a stiff upper lip!"

"Big boys (real men) don't cry!"

Sorry guys, but I beg to differ. By putting our faith in clichés, we are ill prepared for what lies ahead. By "being a man", we may deny the often devastating pain that cancer causes in our wives' bodies and minds—and in our hearts as husbands. Clearly, this is not an effective coping mechanism for the realities of cancer.

Being strong really means accepting that the tears we shed are tears of love—and not a sign of femininity or weakness. Really strong men look beyond the physical and emotional changes our wives experience from tumor growth and treatment side effects and cherish the inner beauty that once made us leave bachelorhood. Physical attraction first brought us together, but inner beauty—the spirit of the women we love—is timeless.

Most men have an extremely difficult time not being in control. However, when cancer invades our marriages, faith in a higher power has to take precedence over machismo and the obsession to control. In fact, by letting go and having faith, cancer can be surmountable. Learning that silence and hugs mean so much more than saying or doing something is crucial to our survival as cancer patients' husbands.

CHAPTER TWO

WRITE ON!

～

My wife was hospitalized for weeks at a time and for a few days on several occasions during her cancer treatment, although much of her care was on an outpatient basis at the Arlington Cancer Center Infusion Center. During one hospitalization, while my wife was in the intensive care unit at Arlington Memorial Hospital, I discovered the therapeutic value of writing. I strongly encourage you to keep a journal during your wife's cancer treatments. Journaling will help you while away the hours during bedside and waiting room vigils and, more importantly, give you a creative outlet for the anxiety we all face when our wives are ill. You may be saying to yourself that you are not a writer. Do not strive for the *New York Times* bestseller list. Your journal is a private document that can help put these surreal days into perspective.

The journal I wrote during my wife's most frightening hospitalization became a short story titled *ICU My Love*. I share it in hopes that it will inspire you to confront your wife's cancer constructively.

ICU My Love

Day One. This story began at 3:15 p.m. on Thursday, September 18, 2003 on a rainy day in Arlington, Texas, a suburb of Dallas. I sat, yellow legal pad and free Compass Bank pen in hand, in the intensive care unit waiting room at Arlington Memorial Hospital. Only a solitary, white-haired, green-smocked volunteer was in the modernly furnished room with me. When I arrived, she was stationed at the compact volunteer desk reading an article in *Reader's Digest*. She did not look up until 15 minutes had passed and her "shift" had come to an end. As she secured her purse carefully tucked out of visitors' reach under the desk, she spoke only to say that she usually stayed until four, but her low blood sugar prohibited another thirty minutes on duty. I told her to "take care" as she exited the room. She said "thanks" and the waiting room became my exclusive domain for a time.

Being alone, having anonymity, when my life is spinning out of control, or in what I call the "surreal zone of family illness", gave me vital time for reflection, to talk with God, and to therapeutically write this essay about a time I begrudgedly accept I cannot control. I wait for news about Robyn, my beloved wife, who suffered kidney and liver failure during her hospitalization for treatment of multiple myeloma and was sent to the ICU. My time at her bedside was unlimited on Station 32, the "cancer floor" where she lived for many weeks when she was progressing well, but being non-responsive and in multi-organ failure makes visitation far more structured and almost unwelcome by some nursing staff.

I have walked alongside Robyn this year on her journey through surgery at St. Luke's Hospital in Houston to replace mitral and aortic heart valves damaged in childhood by

Rheumatic Fever. I have held her hand during weeks of hemodialysis following kidney failure and as she was infused with dozens of intravenous bags of antibiotics and chemotherapy drugs. We have gone from her being bed-bound to walking with a walker hundreds of feet in a leisurely, if not exhausting, walk to recovery from her room to the visitors' waiting room.

Now, as I write these words, she is less than a football field away from me lying in an uneasy slumber on a hospital bed in the high-tech, low-touch ICU. Monitors tracking pulse, respiration, oxygen in the bloodstream, and blood pressure are clearly the priority. Nurses bounce from glass-walled room-to-room viewing monitors and delivering treatments. They occasionally speak.

Not a day has passed since Robyn's medical nightmare began last March that I wished we could have changed places. Quite honestly, I do not know if the roles were reversed that I would have the internal strength necessary to have gone this far. I know my soul mate would be by my side as I have been with her.

This has been a journey of Texas-size proportions. Despite Houston's excellent reputation for medical care, the "cookbook protocol" cancer treatment Robyn started receiving in the Bayou City in May proved totally ineffective. My brother, Andy, a cardiologist and cancer survivor, recommended we entrust Robyn's care to Dr. Karel Dicke at the Arlington Cancer Center. Dr. Dicke, we learned, was a pioneer in the treatment of multiple myeloma. He also was everything Andy described: compassionate, brilliant, upbeat, and Robyn's best hope for remission.

Unfortunately, out of economic necessity, Robyn and I had to be separated during her treatment. My job as a clinic administrator for three prisons in Dayton, Texas, north of Houston, provides the income and health insurance that literally keeps Robyn alive. We have developed a marital bond of phone calls during the week and hospital visitations on weekends. During this ICU stay, I rely on the kindness of my brother and his family for a place to stay.

A family of three large women, likely a mother and her daughters, has entered the waiting room, talking loudly about family matters as if I am not here. They turned on the TV, so my solitude is turned off. Writing is therapeutic and it makes torturous times easier to bear. This essay will surely continue.

Day 2. It is now 4:30 p.m. on Friday. I sit and watch Robyn sleeping soundly in her ICU bed, looking so peaceful. I hold her cold hand—the ICU is kept very cold for some reason—and listen to beeping monitors and a rerun of the *Drew Carey Show* on TV. Robyn's monitor continually tracks her vital signs. Were it not for her swollen extremities and inability to speak or recognize her caregivers or me, the readings on the monitor screen would suggest a vital, healthy woman resting here. I am so afraid that Robyn is going to die. Internally, she is fighting a metabolic disorder that robbed her liver and kidneys of their life-sustaining purposes. I try to rationalize the sheer Hell of an uncertain outcome with knowledge that she is in excellent hands. That God has angels watching over her.

She has come so far! I have tried to be strong. Now, my best efforts to "keep it together," could not keep the floodgate of tears from bursting. I go into a rest room down the hall, lean against the mirror, and cry months of stockpiled tears in a matter of minutes. Big boys do cry! When you love someone as much as I love Robyn, the tears are affirmation of true love—not a sign of weakness or childish behavior. Still, I use the rest room outside the ICU waiting room throughout this day to wipe away the tears. Perhaps tears for me are best shed in solitude.

I did leave my bathroom refuge at one point today to ask God to intervene. I called the holiest friend I know, Rev. Dean Glacken, to give me the words. Even though I was raised as a Jew, I have never known how to truly pray—to ask for God's divine intervention. I reached Dean by cell phone when he and his wife Cheryl (who is fighting breast cancer in Asheville, North Carolina) were at a convention. While the background noise suggested Dean was around many strangers, he asked permission to pray for Robyn and me as if he were standing alongside her ICU bed. He then implored the Almighty to heal Robyn and give me strength. His comfort brought more tears—this time in a hospital hallway—along with a feeling of genuine warmth and restoration of hope.

At 5:00 p.m., I returned to Robyn's room to find an elderly EEG technician carefully combing Robyn's hair, rubber banding her thinning locks, and marking areas of her forehead with a red grease pencil for precise placement of brainwave electrodes. In a strange way, the many hair bands make her look childlike. Perhaps her mother, Inez, banded a young Robyn's hair in the late '50s and early '60s, too. My favorite photo of Robyn is one I carry in my wallet. She is three-years-old in front of a Christmas tree, grinning from ear-to-ear. I often tease people when they ask about my wife by quickly showing them this black and white snapshot.

As I watch the technician focusing on her task, Robyn is unaware of our presence. On the TV screen overlooking her bed is comedian Tim Allen in a rerun of *Home Improvements*. He hits his head on a board. The off-screen audience of "Tool Time" laughs.

All Robyn's electrodes are now in place. The technician

snaps red, white, blue, green, and yellow wires to the computerized EEG machine. She logs onto a laptop computer, turns on a small video camera, and flashes lights on and off to stimulate Robyn's brain activity. The Tool Time canned laughter is now an annoyance, so I turn off the TV and watch the multitude of waves—Robyn's thoughts while she slumbers—on the laptop screen.

Robyn and I spent our first date 11 years ago at a Houston comedy club called Going Bananas. Over the years, we shared so many laughs. How I wish at this moment we could be laughing together about a silly show, the children, the grandchildren—or anything! But she is silent, except for an occasional moan from her chronically dry mouth. The EEG wires remind me of the first time I saw a white woman with corn roll braids. It was in the movie, *Ten*, with Bo Derrick and Dudley Moore. It told the tale of a man obsessed with the ideal woman—a 10. Illness has taking a toll on my beautiful wife, but when I look at her, I see perfection, the woman I adore—and I pray for the true beauty of health to return to her.

Day 5. A new week offers new hope. It is Monday morning, September 22, and while Robyn is still weak and confined to her ICU bed, she is rebounding from the prior week's setbacks. Her daughter, son, father, and brother came to see her over the weekend. When they first arrived, she slept through their visit. Hours later, as we all stood by her bed watching her sleep; she opened her eyes for a moment, spotted her father, and said happily, "Hi, Daddy!" These two words restored our hope and made us laugh again.

When Dr. Doshi, the nephrologist, examined her this morning, I commented to him that Robyn was more alert cognitively—she now knew who we were, yet she turned on and off verbally. Almost on cue, she again opened her eyes, stared at the doctor, and said, "I must have a short." She then dosed off to the background noise of Katie Couric and the *NBC Morning Show*. I stood next to her bed and tried talking to Dr. Doshi, but all I could do was cry. He patted my back, turned, and left the room. Maybe my tears were a short? No. Just true love.

Are you ready to begin your journal? Maybe your wife would like to write down her experiences? The following pages will help you get started.

SUNDAY

MONDAY

TUESDAY

THURSDAY

FRIDAY

_____

_____

_____

_____

_____

_____

_____

_____

_____

_____

_____

_____

_____

_____

_____

_____

_____

_____

_____

_____

_____

SATURDAY

_____

_____

_____

_____

_____

_____

_____

_____

_____

_____

_____

_____

_____

_____

_____

_____

_____

_____

_____

_____

_____

_____

_____

_____

_____

CHAPTER THREE

TO THINE OWN SELF, BE TRUE

❧

To plagiarize the Bard, "To thine own self, be true." Take care of yourself physically, emotionally, spiritually, and financially so you are well prepared to care for your wife. Be prepared to compromise at times on the small things in life—the big thing requiring your energy is your wife's quality of life. Oncologist Karel Dicke told my wife at her first appointment, "Getting well is your full-time job." Learning what is essential and what can be delayed or avoided in your daily life is necessary if you want to help your wife do a job well done and achieve remission. My wife and I were unable to attend her son's wedding since it was held during a course of aggressive chemotherapy. Dr. Dicke said the goal is to see our grandchildren graduate from high school. A good lesson in setting priorities!

I have been fortunate over my wife's first year with cancer to have incredible support from my employer, the University of Texas Medical Branch-Galveston (UTMB) Correctional Managed Care. I was able to transfer from the Houston area to Dallas in order to be closer to my wife. We also have been blessed to have Robyn's father, Bob Porter, living with us in Arlington. Bob is a 78-year-old cancer patient receiving monthly chemotherapy in Houston from Dr. Harry Price, an oncologist who has unquestionably extended Bob's life. Despite Bob's own cancer, he drives Robyn to the infusion center as often as five days a week and cares for her until I arrive home in the evening. As fellow cancer patients, Bob and Robyn understand the good and bad days of treatments and fuel each other's will to live.

I hope you have the support of others to keep you going. If you are your wife's primary caregiver, ask friends or family to give you respite time to take care of yourself. In terms of physical health, schedule an appointment with a family practice or internal medicine physician to have a comprehensive physical exam. Take a daily vitamin and ask the doctor about your taking a baby aspirin and a "statin" pill (Lipitor for example) each day as preventative health measures. If you are "feeling blue" or having difficulty sleeping, talk to your doctor about antidepressants and sleeping pills. Real men do get depressed! Getting a consistent amount of quality sleep each night will help your immune system keep you healthy. Also, consider treating yourself to a massage. You need a little pampering!

Eat a well-balanced diet—fast food at breakfast, lunch and dinner will make you overweight and lethargic. However, occasional "comfort foods"— fried chicken or a decadent hot fudge sundae works for me—are treats for a job well done as a caregiver. Avoid too much caffeine and drink water as often as possible. If you especially enjoy certain types of food—I live for spicy foods—treat yourself. Take pleasure in a good meal. You are worth it.

Exercise—but do not obsess over becoming a health fanatic. Since I really do not like to exercise, my physician in Dallas, Dr. Cynthia Dott, suggested that I use the stairs at work (taking rest stops as needed) instead of the elevator and park far from my destinations to walk more. Walking in a temperature-regulated shopping mall on especially hot or cold days is a form of exercise I have always enjoyed. Unlike an early morning constitutional around your neighborhood, mall walking allows for exercise (often without breaking a sweat) and a healthy dose of people-watching at all times of day. It is very important to be around other people when you are living with cancer in your family. Granted, on some stressful days we want to bury our heads in the sand to get away from it all. And we do need quiet times for introspection. However, I challenge you on these days to do the opposite: be around other people and watch the joy of living on their faces. Even a "terrible" two-year-old having a temper tantrum in the middle of the grocery store demonstrates the vitality of life around us. Watch for a young couple strolling hand-in-hand, perhaps stopping momentarily for a kiss. Remember: this is what we are working towards having back in our lives.

Our emotional well-being is clearly being tested as we walk with our wives on the road to recovery. "Situational depression" is common with many of us. If you do not feel sad, confused, angry, or a sense of hopelessness at this time of your life, then you may be harboring your emotions. Let them out! Help is definitely available through your family doctor, mental health professionals, clergy, and social service agencies. If you are new to your community, contact the local United Way. Many of the agencies they fund offer counseling services on a sliding fee scale. Talk to your friends, other family members or co-workers. They may not understand the depth of your emotional turmoil, but I have found that having someone to vent to can be a great stress reducer.

Thecia Jenkins, a Christian friend, put spiritual wellbeing into four words for me: LET GO, LET GOD. When we accept the fact that a power greater than us alone will ultimately decide our wife's fate, it is a liberating experience. Good oncologists are the earthly hands of God. The oncologists' chemotherapy cocktails and treatment technologies are simply tools of empowerment— gifts from the master healer. Over the past 20 + years that I have worked in health care organizations, when I encountered atheist physicians, I joked to colleagues, "Someone needs to break it to him that M.D. doesn't mean Major Deity." A doctor who understood his place in the grand scheme of things told me a story that I share with you.

A man was standing at the Pearly Gates waiting for St. Peter to escort him into his heavenly home. Suddenly, out of nowhere, a Porsche sped through the gates, causing the man and St. Peter to fall backwards. "Who was that?," asked the man. "Oh, don't mind him. That's God. He thinks he's a doctor."

Have faith, and don't forget to see the lighter side of life— even when everything seems dark and depressing.

It has been said that the best things in life are free. Thank goodness, since cancer care costs can break the bank. We are fortunate enough to have BlueCross and BlueShield health insurance that has covered the lion's share of our family's medical expenses to date. Still, losing a spouse's income causes hardships—but buying "stuff" and paying bills as usual are not high priorities now. If you, like I, are fiscally responsible during normal times, then we have options available to lessen financial stressors. There are non-profit organizations (Consumer Credit Counseling Service-CCCS is a good one in Texas) that work with families like ours to restructure debt without bankruptcy. They negotiate with creditors to lower or waive interest rates and establish consumer-friendly payment plans. Also, most medical providers will accept interest-free payment plans. Tell your wife:

"Honey, it took four years to finance the Honda, it looks like it will take ten to pay for you!" If she has a sense of humor, you'll help her feel better. If not, you'll have more time to walk around the mall.

CHAPTER FOUR

LAUGH OFTEN

‿♢

In a delightful Robin Williams film, medical student Patch Adams clowned around with his patients because the student recognized the healing power of laughter. Faculty members at his medical school were not amused, yet Dr. Adams had the last laugh when, after his training, he was featured in a silver screen biography and incorporated humor into his medical practice.

Physician authors Norman Cousins and Bernie Siegel have written extensively about the healing powers of humor. Dr. Cousins, a cancer survivor, spent many hours watching the Marx Brothers, Three Stooges, and other videos that would tickle his funny bone and release endorphins to stimulate his immune system.

I frequently speak to senior citizen groups and community organizations on healthy living topics and "Laughter is the Best Medicine." During these humorous presentations, I tell true stories that elicit laughs and an occasional groan. Take for example the story of my father that occurred in 2001. He was quite ill with a difficult-to-treat infection. His physician, a well-respected endocrinologist, told me that my father was like a cat with nine lives. Unfortunately, according to the doctor, he was on his last one. How did my father respond? He fired the doctor—and lived three more years! I also give audience members the "Humor Quotient Test" that was developed (tongue-in-cheek) by the University of Texas Health Science Center in Houston. I prescribe it for your wife and you. There is no charge for the exam (other than the cost of this book)! Circle the answer to each question that best describes you. When finished, to score your profile, add up all the a, b, c and d answers on the scorecard at the end of the test. See what your score means by reading the answers that follow.

During an average day, I laugh out loud, snicker or giggle:
A. Once or not at all
B. Two or three times
C. At least once an hour
D. Constantly, it's a sickness.

When I am alone and read, see, or hear something funny, I:
A. Smile to myself
B. Laugh out loud, but look around to see if anyone saw me
C. Laugh out loud and run into the next room to
      share it with someone else
D. Take a shower.

In the past year, I can remember:
A. At least one time I spent a whole minute laughing
B. At least two to five times I spent a whole minute laughing
C. More than five times I spent a whole minute laughing
D. I can't remember. What was the question?

When I'm around other people, they laugh and joke:

A. Never

B. Sometimes

C. Often

D. I never hang around with other people.
      They might laugh at me.

*When faced with daily crises (the dog peed on the rug, you missed
the project deadline, Sally needs brownies for school NOW), I
respond with a laugh:*

A. Never

B. Sometimes

C. Often

D. Only if it's someone else's rug, deadline or child.

*I do things intentionally to make myself laugh (like read the funnies
or listen to comedians):*

A. Never

B. Sometimes

C. Often

D. I can't find the funnies or my television.

The people I spend most of my time with:

A. Leave me feeling drained and depressed

B. Don't really affect my attitude

C. Make me laugh a lot

D. Usually steal my lunch money.

I can name:

A. One thing that almost always makes me laugh

B. Two things that almost always make me laugh

C. At least three things that almost always make me laugh

D. My closest relatives.

I laugh at myself:

A. Never

B. Sometimes

C. Often

D. Only when I'm not in the room.

I do silly things on purpose:

A. Never

B. Sometimes

C. Often

D. On special occasions.

When I hear people laughing at work, the first thing I think is:

A. I wish I could get paid to goof off

B. I wish I knew what the joke is

C. How wonderful that they're having a good time

D. That it's Saturday and I shouldn't even be here!

Total # of A's __ x 0 = 0 points

Total # of B's __ x 1 = ___ pts

Total # of C's __ x 2 = ___ pts

Total # of D's __ x 3 = ___ pts

Total points (A + B + C + D) = _____

What this all means:

Score of 0-5: You are suffering from humor malnutrition. Even your funny bone is sad. Your case is so serious that you may actually need a humor transplant if you don't do something quick! Start today! Crack a smile, tickle your funny bone, practice laughing at home, and find a friend who can teach you how to laugh at life and yourself.

Score of 6-10: You occasionally have a good laugh, but laughter is like exercise. You have to do it regularly to get the full benefit. Use it or lose it! Start talking to squirrels, making up limericks, wearing weird earrings. You've made a good start, now really lighten up!

Score of 11-20: You are humorously fit! Not only do you approach life with the right amount of humor and benefit from it, but you also make others' lives more enjoyable. Get out there and teach those people who can't seem to laugh.

Score of 21-33: Now, you're downright silly, aren't you? Don't stifle that childish instinct! Sure they told you in school that the class clown would never go anywhere in life. But, they were wrong! Remember Milton Berle, Bob Hope and George Burns? They lived long lives...laughing all the way to the bank.

CHAPTER FIVE

THERE ARE NO STUPID QUESTIONS

༄

Have you ever not asked a question because you thought it was "stupid"? I ask you this question because I am naturally inquisitive and spent three years working as a journalist before entering the health care field. I ask a lot of questions. I still may preface what I ask with, "May I ask a stupid question?" or "I can't help but ask…". As most of our elementary school teachers once said, "There are no stupid questions." Especially when your wife has cancer. So ask away!

During my father's final years, I went with him to doctors' appointments and was impressed that he carried with him a list of the many medications he was taking, a diary of glucometer readings tracking his glucose levels, and at least a half-dozen questions. He would not let the doctors leave their exam rooms until he had answers to every question. Once, when my father was hospitalized in an intensive care unit, I asked the nurse what was in the IV bag she was hanging. I told her I was concerned since my Dad was diabetic. While answering my question, she realized she was infusing an incorrect bag, quickly removed it, and thanked me for bringing this to her attention.

Prior to my wife's multiple myeloma diagnosis, she went

into kidney failure and required hemodialysis three times a week. While receiving a blood transfusion at the hospital in Houston during one dialysis session, she suddenly had great difficulty breathing, her blood pressure skyrocketed, and she became incoherent. Fortunately, her nephrologist, Dr. Mario Rubin, was writing in a chart just outside her room and quickly responded. As I sat at her bedside, I started asking what was going on. Did she need more oxygen? The doctor very calmly gave an order, which the nurse dutifully followed. He then very firmly asked me to go to the waiting room. In retrospect, I learned that there is clearly a time and a place to ask questions— and during an emergency is not the time. However, from this experience, and speaking with Dr. Rubin later that day, I learned that my wife needs to be pre-medicated with 25 milligrams of Benadryl prior to receiving blood and platelets, and the slower the rate of infusion, the better it is tolerated. Since her cancer care has required numerous infusions, this has proven very important.

As the husband of a cancer patient, you probably have many questions that you have hesitated to ask. Dr. Dicke and his nurse practitioner, Sylvia Hanks, in office appointments, at the infusion center and hospital, have made me feel like a vital member of the care team by very kindly answering all the questions I ask and including Robyn and me in treatment planning. My advice to you—if your wife's doctors and nurses do not fully answer your questions in layman's terms, either 1) keep asking verbally or in writing, or 2) find another doctor. Here are a few questions you might consider:

How many patients have you treated for this type of cancer?

May I contact two or three of these patients? (Health care privacy laws require physicians to first ask other patients if they wish to be contacted).

What, if any, are the side effects of her treatment?

Are there any foods or drinks she should avoid?

What time of day should she take this medicine? With or without food?

Is it okay to take vitamins or herbal remedies while undergoing treatment?

What will the treatment schedule be?

What are signs or symptoms of problems I should be aware of during and following treatments?

Are there any new medications or drug trials available?

May some of her treatments be delivered at home?

How will we know if she is improving?

Will you tell us if she is unlikely to recover?

Do you refer patients to Hospice?

There are likely dozens of other questions that will come to mind on your journey through cancer treatment and recovery. Asking questions will enable you to objectively evaluate each new situation and to be a real support to the health care providers and your wife. Knowledge is power and a comfort too!

CHAPTER SIX

REDEFINING YOUR MARRIAGE

⟳

A s a man working in health care, I am often asked if I am a doctor. My answer is usually, "no, but I play one on TV." However, since my wife has been treated for cancer for some time now, I may be able to become an "honorary" nurse (if not a doctor). I have learned how to infuse total parenteral nutrition (TPN) through an intravenous (IV) line at home, flush vascular catheters with saline and Heparin, do dressing changes and basic wound care, dispense medications, and other tasks that have enabled my wife to spend a minimal amount of time in the hospital, have fewer infections, and enjoy more time with our children and grandchildren. Accumulating and detailing these technical skills seems rather impersonal when writing about my beloved wife, especially since she has told me on numerous occasions that I could teach other men how to be good husbands.

However, as our wives go through the stages of cancer—discovery, treatment, and God-willing recovery, our roles as husbands definitely change. Men who never did house cleaning or cooking suddenly become Mr. Clean and Emeril (at least in spirit). Childcare and children's after-school activities that were once shared responsibilities are now clearly on the husband's daily agenda. For many of us, through the treatment periods, passionate sex becomes snuggling, tender kisses and back rubs. For my wife and me, this tenderness is very gratifying—and we look forward to full intimacy when health allows.

Cancer treatment is unquestionably one of the most stressful times in our individual and familial lives. There are essentially two options available to us: 1) channel the stress constructively, or 2) distress. I encourage the first and strongly suggest you find ways not to do the latter. Here are a few stress management ideas to consider.

Talk to a social worker, marriage and family therapist, or psychologist and ask them to teach you effective stress management techniques. Your wife's oncologist will likely know of mental health professionals that are attuned to families facing cancer. The American Cancer Society also has resources.

Check with your employer to see if they offer an Employee Assistance Program (EAP). These counselors have printed resources that they can send to your home and often will have supportive sessions with you over the phone or in person that are free or very low cost.

Do not forget to celebrate whenever possible. When my wife celebrated her 48th birthday in the hospital, we toasted the occasion with cups of "sparkling" Sprite and ate her favorite shrimp dinner ordered take-out from Outback. On the Valentine's Day after my wife's diagnosis, we attended a dinner and show at a small town country club. We dressed up and forgot about the cancer for a few hours.

Have as many movie nights as possible. Rent videotapes or DVDs, buy Good and Plenty or chocolate-covered raisins, make popcorn, then lay back and escape into Hollywood fantasies.

Take a trip to see family or friends—or no one in particular. A weekend drive and lunch at a "discovered" café may be more budget-friendly than that trip to Paris you had planned for some day. But follow the road wherever it takes you. If friends and family are important to your wife, as they are to us, make time to see them or ask them to come visit.

Use email and the telephone to stay in touch with friends who really know what to say. We have an email list of friends and family I named "Robyn Supporters" and I keep these people updated about our life on at least a monthly basis. Many of them respond with prayers, good news about new babies and other joyous times, funny stories, and other uplifting escapes from our cancer reality. I have a few close friends who allow me to vent my anger and frustration over my wife's cancer. Most often, it is not what they say that reduces my stress level, but that they really listen.

Finally, learn to daydream. There is a relaxation technique called creative visualization that can be very relaxing. Purchase audiotapes or write and read scripts to your wife of relaxing scenarios while she sits or lays comfortably with her eyes closed.

These seven ideas should help reduce the stress that is a daily component of our lives with cancer. By no means is this an inclusive list, and I encourage you to find other things that you can do together (or alone when you need a break) to relax and enjoy each day's gift of life.

Try this creative visualization escape today. It is my stress-relieving present to you.

We are driving slowly down a country road. It's a beautiful day. About 70 degrees. No humidity to speak of. The sky is a brilliant blue. Not a cloud can be seen. Two large black birds circle above us. We roll down the windows. Country-fresh air wisps across our faces. The view outside is so relaxing. So different from our usual commutes. Lining both sides of the two-lane road are fields of corn that seem to go on forever. Rows and rows of bright green corn stalks. A scarecrow with overalls and a straw hat is mounted high above the field on our right. A crow sits on the scarecrow's straw-filled shoulder unaware that he is supposed to be afraid. On our left, an elderly farmer is driving a John Deere tractor up one row and down the other. As we continue down this restful country road, we see a field plush with wildflowers. The blue, red, orange and white blossoms blow gently in the wind. On the edge of this canvas of brilliant colors sits a solitary picnic table. We turn the car off the paved road and onto a gravel one. We park, open the trunk, and take out a wicker picnic basket. We walk, hand-in-hand, over to the picnic table, and sit down for a spell. We're hungry from our country journey. Inside the basket is fried chicken, biscuits, creamy cole slaw, and a pecan pie. As we enjoy this wonderful meal, we stare into each others eyes and say...I love you darling.

CHAPTER SEVEN

PARENTING AND CANCER

❦

I was 29-years-old when my mother died from cancer. Old enough to know what cancer was, but not old enough to lose a mother. Are we ever old enough to lose someone we love? Not a day goes by that I do not think of my mother. Did this loss prepare me for my wife's cancer? Did the losses you had in your life make your wife's cancer any easier to bear? My mother left me with many happy memories—she was the artistic parent in our home: a gifted pianist, kind and giving, the inspiration for my creative writing endeavors—and she lived a good life for over 50 years (nearly 11 years between her mastectomies and the cancer that killed her). Her battle with cancers helped me understand the importance of seeing each day as a gift. As my wife and I share her cancer journey, we appreciate and value each day we are given. We exchange "I love you" comments and kisses frequently. We try to make each day as normal as possible— especially for our children (who are nearly 300 miles away).

Robyn and I are a "blended" family. Her daughter, Nicole, is 26-years-old and son, Jason, is 22. They are married, the parents of four children, and live near each other in a small community south of Houston. While they now have very busy lives as young adults, they are very close to their mother. Nicole calls daily to share stories of grandson Carson and other news to keep Robyn informed, and often entertained. They have a very special mother-daughter bond, and Nicole feels her mother's pain and, by staying in touch, demonstrates there is so very much to live for. Jason, the more introverted child, stays informed through his sister and occasional calls, but his love and concern for his mother are genuine. They, and I, have many plans for their mother's future. Robyn's father and I try to keep them informed of changes in her medical condition. While we believe that only God knows when her last breath will be, sharing the good news and the bad with her children is clearly the right thing to do. There is not a one-size-fits-all approach to talking to your children about your wife's cancer. However, on-going communication keeps hope alive and gives the children some perspective on the future.

My children, Nathan, age 16, and Benjamin, age 13, live with their mother in Houston. Nathan and Benjamin love and respect their stepmother, but are not very close to her. However, when she was diagnosed with multiple myeloma, Nathan did an Internet search and gave us sites with far more information than was available from her Houston oncologist. He even shared news of Velcade, a promising new drug approved by the Food and Drug Administration (FDA). Dr. Dicke hopes to use Velcade as Robyn's maintenance therapy. Death is not a foreign concept to my sons. They experienced the loss of their maternal grandmother a few years ago and their paternal grandfather in 2004. They fully understand how painful cancer can be, and I know they were a comfort to their mother when Grandma Renee finally succumbed to cancer. They were a comfort to me following my father's death.

When speaking to my sons, I share the facts, as well as my

pain and fear with them, hoping, as with Nicole and Jason, that the knowledge will give them strength and prepare them for whatever comes next. More importantly, I want them to see what sacrifices we make for the one we love—hoping this example of love will enable them to be compassionate husbands and loving men.

Before Robyn's illness, while we lived in Houston, we saw all of the children and grandchildren regularly. While we love them all dearly, Robyn's recovery from cancer had to be our #1 priority. Cancer usurped the lion's share of my wife's energy— but the sound of her children's and grandchildren's voices always elicits a smile.

My advice for your children:

Talk openly and honestly with them about your wife's cancer in age-appropriate terms. Answer the questions they ask to the best of your ability.

For young children, visit the library, bookstores or counseling centers to acquire books on children and loss.

Schedule time with your children alone and as a family during the months of cancer care.

If they fear that Mom will die, explain the cycle of life and death to them. Young children may also fear that you will die too and leave them alone. Try to comfort them.

Contact the counselors at your children's schools to make them aware of what your family is going through. Ask them to let you know if your children "act out" or have changes in behavior. These are signs that mental health care may be needed. The school counselors often can recommend appropriate professionals. They also may be able to give you the names and phone numbers of other families that have young children and understand life with cancer.

Cry with your children, hold them, comfort them, and say "I love you" often. They will help you on this journey perhaps as much as you help them.

In conclusion, we have all heard the folklore (or fact) that men refuse to ask for directions—even when traveling in unknown territories. Now is not the time to wander aimlessly. If you are lost in dealing with your wife's cancer—especially when communicating with your children—STOP, and ask for directions.

CHAPTER EIGHT

WHEN REMISSION ISN'T POSSIBLE

◦✍◦

"You win some, you lose some." "It's not important whether you win or lose, it's how you play the game." These sports adages we grew up believing seem really ridiculous at this time in our lives. Our reality is: if our wives achieve remission, we won. Game over. Pack up the car, we're going home.

For us, on a personal level, losing to cancer—even though we played the game with the greatest finesse—means death. On a spiritual level, Christians, Jews and others of faith, believe death can be a beautiful thing. It is the end of suffering and a time for heavenly rest. They find solace in the Twenty-third Psalm:

The Lord is my shepherd; I shall not want.

He makes me to lie down in green pastures; He leads me in the paths of righteousness for His name's sake.

Yea, though I walk through the valley of the shadow of death, I will fear no evil; for You are with me; Your rod and your staff, they comfort me.

You prepare a table before me in the presence of my enemies; You anoint my head with oil; My cup runs over.

Surely goodness and mercy shall follow me all the days of my life; and I will dwell in the house of the Lord forever.

If your wife survives—as so many people with cancer do today—I hope you realize the priceless gift your family has received. Celebrate!

If your wife's condition is terminal, I hope the preceding seven chapters provided some comfort and guidance. Once you are told that treatment is no longer effective, it is time to ask the oncologist to estimate your wife's remaining life. While this may seem insensitive or morbid, it is something you need to know. If the doctor believes your wife has six months or less to live, contact a Hospice organization in your community immediately.

It is important to realize that oncologists can only estimate remaining life based on their experience and the patient's current health status. Patients have been known to live longer than projected (when they maintain a strong will to live and continue receiving supportive care) or fewer days (when they believe death is imminent).

As a former Hospice administrator, I assure you the angels of mercy (nurses, nursing assistants, social workers, counselors and chaplains) that are drawn to this field are outstanding. They are trained in palliative (comfort) care and serve your family's medical, emotional and spiritual needs. All offer bereavement services and many sponsor support groups for children.

Time is of the essence, as Hospice staff will address your wife's pain and be a support for your family until her final breath. Unfortunately, in America, Hospice referrals too often are made when the patient has only a few days or weeks to live. Medicare and most insurance plans support Hospice over the final six months. Also, under the Family and Medical Leave Act (FMLA), many employers must protect your job and benefits while you spend this essential time with your wife.

As all of us near the end of life, there is "unfinished business" that Hospice professionals believe must be completed before we die in peace. When you and your wife spend time together in her final days, try to listen more than you talk. When you do speak, gently guide her in completing unfinished business. Consider these examples:

Does she need to apologize to someone she feels she treated unfairly?

Does she need to write or speak to a friend or family member to say goodbye?

Does she need to travel to a favorite vacation spot one last time?

Does she need to meet with a lawyer to write her will?

Does she need assurance that you (and the children) will be okay when she dies?

When my wife's grandmother died under Hospice care in Nebraska, her nurse described the time leading up to her peaceful death as "opening the door." She said her goodbyes to friends and neighbors, summoned her children from Colorado, North Carolina and Texas so they could be with her, made sure all her obligations were met, stopped eating and only drank sips of water, then laid down for her final rest.

CHAPTER NINE

MY EARTHLY ANGEL
HAS A NEW HEAVENLY HOME

⁀৹

O n Thursday, March 18, 2004, at 10:30 p.m., nearly one hour after I fell asleep, the phone at my bedside rang. It was a nurse from the telemetry unit at Arlington Memorial Hospital: "Your wife is having trouble breathing. She asked me to call you. She needs you here. We're on our way to the CCU!" Ten minutes later, I was at her bedside in telemetry as the staff transferred oxygen and monitors to portable units for the ride down the hall. I kissed her on the forehead, held her hand, and did not let go until she arrived in the coronary care unit.

Her blood was not getting enough oxygen to feed her vital organs. At 4:00 a.m. on Friday, March 19, 2004, her CCU nurse, Royce, called me out into the hall: "Your wife needs to be put on a ventilator." Robyn and I had discussed whether either of us would choose to be placed on life support if faced with this decision. At the time, we both said, "NO!" I asked Royce to call my brother Andy, a cardiologist, brief him, and ask for his thoughts on ventilating Robyn. Up until this point, I was able to make many decisions with and for Robyn. When facing this life-or-death reality, I could not make this decision alone. Andy, kindly and calmly, told me that Robyn definitely should go on the vent and the next 48-hours would be crucial. A time-line for life or death! My grief and fear became overwhelming. My tears flowed freely. A nurse gently rubbed my back to comfort me.

Ironically, in retrospect, Robyn faced a similar crisis with her mother. She, along with her father and brother, had to make the ventilator decision for her mother, Inez, as she was in an emergency room dying of emphysema several years ago. They had the courage—guided by Joel Reed, a truly empathetic pulmonologist, to make the decision to allow her to die gracefully.

I sat at Robyn's bedside to ask her again whether she would allow a ventilator to be used, if only for the short-term. She softly said, "no." With two nurses witnessing her wishes, then leaving the room, I tearfully asked my love: "Are you sure?" "Yes," she assured me, then inquired, "what will happen if I don't?" I looked at a nurse standing in the doorway and she frowned. "Honey, you will die if you don't get on a vent." As I clutched her hand—unsuccessfully trying not to cry—she agreed to be placed first on a continuous air pressure machine (C-Pap), and if needed, a ventilator.

Then, our world was turned upside down. Moments after being connected to the C-Pap, she went into cardiac arrest. I stood in a corner, trembling yet frozen in the moment, shocked by the words bellowing from Robyn's room throughout the CCU: "Code Blue CCU 17. Code Blue CCU 17." A swarm of doctors, nurses, respiratory therapists and other staff entered her room. One man disconnected the C-Pap, while another took a CPR bag from the wall and began pumping air into her deflated lungs. Two nurses aggressively did chest compressions while others felt and listened for a pulse. Then one nurse yelled, "I have a pulse.

I have a strong pulse!" Robyn was with us again; and as she was intubated and placed on a ventilator, a sense of calm returned.

At 1:00 p.m., I told Robyn I was going to walk to a nearby restaurant for a bite to eat. In acknowledging my hunger pangs, she squeezed my hand, winked and smiled lovingly, as if to say, "Have a good lunch!" At 1:30 p.m., I returned to her room to find my lifeless wife stretched out in her hospital bed. The doctors tried to wean her from the ventilator to the C-Pap. She had another cardiac arrest—this time CPR failed to revive her heart in time to adequately feed her brain. She was being placed back on the ventilator as I entered the room. I grabbed her hand, squeezed it, looked into her dilated eyes and cried: "Honey, can you hear me?" Her spirit clearly was gone.

After talking again with Andy and the pulmonologist, the only option remaining was to allow Robyn's children, brother and father time to say goodbye. The ventilator was breathing for her and could sustain "life" for necessary grieving time. Within a couple of hours, her daughter, Nicole, and son, Jason, were at her bedside. My co-workers from UTMB came to lend their support. My brother, Andy, and his wife, Andrea, as well as three ministers were there to support us in our mourning. By 10:00 p.m., her father and brother arrived.

By 10:30 p.m., with the ventilator disconnected, my earthly angel, Robyn, departed from our world to be with God. According to her oncologist, the multiple myeloma spread to her heart. While the chemotherapy and stem cell transplant had been effective in slowly rebuilding Robyn's white blood cells, pharmaceuticals and self-donated cells could not prevent the heart damage that ultimately took her last breath.

Watching her die will be emblazoned in my heart and mind until the day I leave this world. Having the opportunity to care for her throughout this mind-boggling journey was a gift. I was taught that each day and true love must be cherished—because they are fleeting things. Thank you, Robyn, for the love and lessons.

WEBSITES

The following organizations' websites are wonderful resources for families living with cancer. For assistance in your community, contact the Education, Case Management or Social Work departments at your hospital, or consult with your oncologist or family physician.

American Association for Marriage & Family Therapists	www.aamft.org
American Cancer Society	www.cancer.org
Arlington Cancer Center	www.acctx.com
Hospice Foundation of America	www.hospicefoundation.org
International Myeloma Foundation	www.myeloma.org
Susan B. Komen Breast Cancer Foundation	www.komen.org
Leukemia & Lymphoma Society	www.leukemia.org
Mayo Clinic	www.mayoclinic.com
Memorial Sloan-Kettering Cancer Center	www.mskcc.org

Multiple Myeloma Research Foundation	www.multiplemyeloma.org
National Association of Social Workers	www.socialworkers.org
National Cancer Institute	www.cancer.gov
National Center for Grieving Children & Families	www.grievingchild.org
National Cervical Cancer Coalition	www.nccc-online.org
National Hospice & Palliative Care Organization	www.nhpco.org
National Ovarian Cancer Coalition	www.ovarian.org
Society of Gynecologic Oncologists	www.sgo.org
UT MD Anderson Cancer Center	www.mdanderson.org
United Way of America	www.national.unitedway.org/myuw

ABOUT THE AUTHOR

Mark Elliott Miller was born on August 10, 1960 in Houston, Texas, and has lived in Texas and North Carolina. A former photojournalist and current health care administrator, Mr. Miller earned a Bachelor of Science degree in professional writing from the University of Houston–Downtown and a Master of Public Health degree from the University of North Carolina at Chapel Hill. He also received training as a nursing facility administrator from San Jacinto College in Pasadena, Texas and as an eldercare ombudsman (advocate) from the University of Texas Health Science Center in Houston, Texas.

He is the author of numerous articles and two books, *Extraordinary Encounters In An Ordinary Life* in 2002, and *Advice for Life from the Mouths of Elders, One Hundred Ways To Grow Old Gracefully* in 2003. An accomplished public speaker and award-winning Toastmaster, Mr. Miller enjoys speaking to groups on living with vitality, laughter and healing, and other inspirational topics.

Since the 1980's, Mr. Miller has served as a volunteer board member for the American Cancer Society, American Red Cross, ALS Association, Fort Bend County Mental Health Association, Morganton-Burke County Senior Center, and Senior Services Alliance. He has also volunteered for United Way and the University of Texas Health Science Center–Houston Ombudsman Program.

Mr. Miller may be reached through his website, www.mark elliottmiller.com or by e-mail at angelsquillproductions@yahoo.com.

READERS' COMMENTS

"You make the reader feel that he or she is sharing your experience on every page. Your advice about humor and laughter is right on target. Your advice on stress management as well as advice for children is thoughtful and helpful. Your listing of websites will be useful to many patients." — *Robert A. Kyle, MD, The Mayo Clinic, Rochester, Minnesota*

"A valuable resource for caregivers." — *Susie Novis, President, International Myeloma Foundation, North Hollywood, California*

"What a wonderful and real manuscript! It speaks to my heart and I know it will to patients and families. Great." — *Jan Garza, Oncology Nurse Specialist, St. Luke's Episcopal Hospital, Houston, Texas*

"It's very personal, very practical, loving and things guys will relate." — *Chava White, LMSW-ACP, Oncology Social Worker / Case Manager, St. Luke's Episcopal Hospital, Houston, Texas*

Share your strategies for living with cancer or comments about this book and they may be posted on the www.markelliottmiller.com website. If you are living with cancer, or cancer in the past has changed your life forever, then your thoughts may help others now on a similar journey.

Mail your comments to:

Mark Elliott Miller
835 East Lamar Blvd., #357, Arlington, Texas 76011

visit: www.markelliottmiller.com

e-mail: angelsquillproductions@yahoo.com

Printed in the United Kingdom by
Lightning Source UK Ltd., Milton Keynes
139550UK00001B/14/A